Careers in Pharmacy

Edited by

Brenda Ecclestone

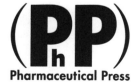

Pharmaceutical Press

Published by the Pharmaceutical Press
1 Lambeth High Street, London SE1 7JN

First edition 1998

© 1998 Pharmaceutical Press

Cover design by Interbrand Newell & Sorrell, London
Text design by Barker/Hilsdon, Lyme Regis, Dorset
Typeset by Photoprint, Torquay, Devon
Printed in Great Britain by TJ International, Padstow, Cornwall

ISBN   0 85369 409 5

A catalogue record for this book is available from the British
Library.

Careers in Pharmacy

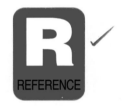

Contents

Contributors

Barry Andrews *Community pharmacy*

Malcolm Bayly *Community pharmacy*

Alison Blenkinsopp *Returning to work*

Michael Burden *The preregistration year*

Sarah Cockbill *Further career options (agricultural and veterinary pharmacy)*

Valda Elson *The career break* and *Maternity leave*

Angela Fell *Pharmaceutical advisers and community services pharmacists*

Katy Fitzsimon *Industrial pharmacy*

Rosalind Grant *Pharmaceutical advisers and community services pharmacists*

Cathy Harrington *Industrial pharmacy*

Gillian Hawksworth *Community pharmacy*

Jeannette Howe *Further career options (The Civil Service)*

Mark Koziol *Locum pharmacy*

Ann Lewis *Hospital pharmacy*

Millicent Martin   *The job application*

Pamela Mason   *Further career options (journalism and editorial work)*

Catherine McClelland   *Education*

Jane Nicholson   *Industrial pharmacy*

Rose Marie Parr   *Returning to work*

Hannah Rees   *Hospital pharmacy*

Kay Roberts   *Further career options (The Civil Service)*

Jane Sheridan   *Education*

Katrina Simister   *Hospital pharmacy*

David Temple   *Returning to work*

Tee Treacy   *Further career options (The Prison Pharmaceutical Service)*

Pamela Warrington   *Further career options (The Civil Service)*

Nicholas Wood   *Community pharmacy*

Preface

Careers in Pharmacy has evolved from the information pack developed by the National Association of Women Pharmacists (NAWP) entitled the *Women in Pharmacy Pack*.

Careers in Pharmacy provides guidance to all pharmacists and pharmacy students; in particular, those who are embarking on their career or returning to pharmacy practice after a career break.

The initial chapters on job applications and the preregistration year include information on compilation of the curriculum vitae, interview technique, preregistration training, and the preregistration examination.

Subsequent chapters give an overview of careers that are relevant to the pharmacist, including community pharmacy, hospital pharmacy, industrial pharmacy, education, locum pharmacy, pharmaceutical advisers and community services pharmacists, and further career options. These chapters should not be considered as detailed accounts but are intended to give guidance when making career choices. The chapters were contributed by practising pharmacists.

The career break and its implications are examined, followed by a chapter that discusses returning to work, which addresses the need for re-training and reviews flexible working and childcare arrangements. Finally, there is a chapter on benefits and rights when taking maternity leave.

The Pharmaceutical Press is pleased to acknowledge the contribution to this project of the NAWP and all those involved in the preparation of the original *Women in Pharmacy Pack*, particularly Christine Glover, Pat Hoare, and Constance Lady Perris. Millicent Martin is thanked for her assistance in revising the text for publication, along with Anne Edwards for her secretarial skills.

The job application

The search for employment can be daunting, particularly for those looking for their first job, or returning to work after a lengthy absence. The quality of a candidate's job application and the way the candidate presents themselves at interview are both vital to the chance of securing a post. There follows some general guidance about job searching and the preparation of job applications; more detailed advice can be found in specialised publications.

Many job vacancies for pharmacists are advertised in *The Pharmaceutical Journal* (published weekly by the Royal Pharmaceutical Society of Great Britain and sent to all registered pharmacists) and the *Chemist and Druggist*. In addition, the broadsheet, and some local newspapers may carry advertisements for pharmacists.

THE CURRICULUM VITAE

A prospective employer gains their first impression of a candidate from the curriculum vitae and based on this, the employer will assess the suitability of the applicant for the position. The employer will wish to ascertain that the candidate's qualifications are adequate and that the candidate will perform well in the job and fit into the existing team.

Both the curriculum vitae and covering letter should be tailored to suit the job. It is becoming more common for applicants to summarise their key capabilities and strengths in a 'profile' section on the opening sheet of the curriculum vitae. The curriculum vitae should be clear and concise. Ideally, it should fit on two sides of A4 paper. Ensure that a clear font style and a simple layout is used and that the information provided is consistent and that the spelling is accurate.

Although it is expected that the curriculum vitae should mainly include academic and professional achievements, a pharmacist returning to work following a career break should emphasise any skills acquired during that period.

The following framework may be useful as a guide to writing a curriculum vitae (the information should be in reverse chronological sequence):

....

Name

Personal details
   Address (include full postcode)
   Telephone number (daytime and/or evening)
   Date of birth
   Marital status
   Nationality

Profile
   Summarise key capabilities and strengths; be succinct.

Main achievements
   Highlight strengths.

Education
   List universities, colleges, and secondary schools attended with dates of attendance.

Qualifications

List all qualifications, with dates and grades, gained from secondary school onwards, including any vocational qualifications.

Mention any projects undertaken during either the undergraduate or postgraduate period. These may be discussed at interview, so familiarity with your work is essential.

Career profile

Start with the most recent position, be concise, and state:

Name of employer(s)   Position held   Dates

Do not omit information for a particular timespan, the interviewer will inevitably enquire further about that period.

Additional information

For example:

- membership of professional bodies or relevant committees;
- conferences or postgraduate courses attended;
- list any publications that you have written (if the number exceeds six, write the full references on a separate sheet as an appendix);
- sporting interests and hobbies;
- any posts held in local organisations.

References

You may wish to include names, titles and full addresses of two or three referees at the end of the curriculum vitae. Alternatively, you may wish to state that referees will be made available on request. Ask permission from your referees in advance and advise them that they may be asked to supply a reference for a particular position.

The information on the curriculum vitae will be referred to at the interview. Do not be tempted to exaggerate anything.

THE INTERVIEW

The success of a job application can often depend upon the degree of preparation devoted to the interview. It is likely that the employer has spent considerable time and effort planning the interview; the interviewer will expect a similar effort from the applicant.

Before the interview, try to obtain some company literature and read it thoroughly. Anticipate potential questions and prepare suitable answers. If appropriate, make an informal telephone call to ascertain further details of the post, the organisation, and working conditions. Establish the exact location of where the interview will be held, and consider the availability of public transport or car parking. Write a positive letter confirming the interview arrangements.

Keep a copy of the original application and the job description and be familiar with both before the interview. Write down any relevant questions you have which should be short and not too numerous. In particular, try to think about special skills or experience that comply with the job specification, and which may gain you an advantage over other candidates. In addition, identify areas of experience that fall short of the specification and consider positive responses that will convince the interviewer that any apparent lack of skill or experience can be overcome.

An awareness of topical issues within the profession is essential. Read recent pharmaceutical literature to familiarise yourself with current topics and key issues. At the interview, wear appropriate, clean, comfortable clothes. Presentation is important; the candidate's outward appearance is the first impression gained by the interviewer. Arrive early for the interview to allow time to relax. On entering the interview room, try to look confident, relaxed, and alert; offer a short, but firm handshake.

The first minutes of an interview can be crucial. After a few introductory questions, the interviewer will begin to ask more searching questions to appraise the candidate's technical skill and knowledge, and to assess whether the candidate is suited to the position.

During the interview, after listening carefully to a question it is a good idea to take a thoughtful pause before replying. In addition, when a reply to a question is considered to be complete, there is no need to say more; allow a moment of silence, giving the interviewer a chance to enquire further or to go on to the next question. Smile frequently and maintain eye contact with the interviewer. Try to avoid tentative language, for example phrases such as 'I feel. . .' or 'think. . .'.

Listed below are some common interview questions; it is advisable to prepare answers to these in advance of the interview:

Common interview questions

Tell me about yourself/your expertise/your experience.

Why did you choose pharmacy as a career? Was it a good choice?

How would you fulfil the job description?

Do you have a career plan?

How does your career to date comply with your plan?

How does this post comply with your plan?

Why are you interested in this position?

What motivates you?

What are your strengths and weaknesses, especially with respect to this position?

Do you work well as part of a team/on your own?

Why did you leave your last job? (Try to be constructive.)

What are your ambitions for the next five years?

The candidate will normally be given the opportunity to ask questions at the end of the interview; this is the chance to clarify any points relating to the post, the organisation, or the terms and conditions of employment offered. However, consider these questions carefully; do not ask anything that may jeopardise any chance of securing the post. When the interview has finished, ask what happens next, and when. Finally, remember that all candidates are open to scrutiny from the minute they arrive at the interview location until the minute they leave.

FURTHER INFORMATION

Bolles RN. *The 1997 What Color is your Parachute: A Practical Manual for Job Hunters and Career Changers.* Berkeley: Ten Speed Press, 1997.

Eggert M. *The Perfect Interview.* London: Century Business, 1992.

Forbes D. How to secure a post. *Br J Pharm Pract.* 1990;12(1): 8,10.

Miller Freeman. *Chemist & Druggist.* Tonbridge: Miller Freeman.

Parents at Work – A Practical Guide for Parents Returning to Work. London: Parents at Work, 1995.

Royal Pharmaceutical Society of Great Britain. *The Pharmaceutical Journal.* London: Pharmaceutical Press.

Wallis M. *Getting There – Job Hunting for Women.* London: Kogan Page Ltd, 1990.

USEFUL ADDRESSES

**Equal Opportunities
Commission**
Publicity Section
Overseas House
Quay Street
Manchester M3 3HN

Parents at Work
Murray House
Beech Street
London
EC2Y 8AD
Telephone: 0171 628 3578

2

The preregistration year

All pharmacy graduates intending to register as pharmacists are required to complete satisfactorily a one-year period of preregistration training. The preregistration programme is designed to assist the trainee to apply the knowledge gained during academic studies and to develop that knowledge along with the skills required in professional practice.

For many undergraduates the successful completion of the degree examinations may be seen as the most significant hurdle in the path to becoming a pharmacist. However, it is essential that before embarking on the final undergraduate year pharmacy students should carefully consider the options available to them with regard to their preregistration training.

CHOICE OF PHARMACY SECTOR

The preregistration year can be undertaken in any of the three main branches of pharmacy, although at least six months must be spent in either the community or hospital sector. Pharmacy graduates who wish to undertake part of their preregistration training in the pharmaceutical industry must undertake a programme of joint experience, organised between the pharmaceutical company and either a hospital or community pharmacy. The joint programme must be approved by the Royal Pharmaceutical Society of Great Britain (RPSGB) before commencement.

Students who have a clear idea of their preferred field of practice should use their preregistration training as an opportunity to progress in their chosen sector. Information should be requested from prospective employers and advice may also be sought from pharmacists already working in the field. Attendance at local branch meetings of the RPSGB presents an opportunity for discussion with experienced pharmacists.

Students are advised to read the *Code of Practice for Preregistration Recruitment* published by the RPSGB. This document outlines the Royal Pharmaceutical Society Council's view of best practice in the recruitment of pharmacy students for preregistration training posts. It states the responsibilities of both the student and the employer.

The British Pharmaceutical Students Association (BPSA) offers advice about training places. The BPSA was established in 1942 to represent undergraduate students and preregistration graduates. The aim of the organisation is to promote the welfare of members by encouraging and facilitating the interchange of ideas and opinions between members and by providing a platform for communication with other pharmaceutical organisations. In 1986, the BPSA appointed a Graduate Officer to promote the welfare of pharmacy trainees. Preregistration trainees receive a regular newsletter entitled *Graduate Link* to keep them informed about developments within the BPSA. There is also an annual preregistration conference.

THE PREREGISTRATION TUTOR

Every preregistration training establishment must be approved by the RPSGB. One of the requirements for approval is that a full-time preregistration tutor works on the premises. The tutor must have been registered as a pharmacist for at least three years and must also meet the targets set by the Council of the RPSGB with regard to postgraduate continuing education. The tutor is required to lead by example and to serve as a learning resource by answering questions, providing feedback, and guiding the trainee as appropriate. The tutor should also ensure that there is continuity in the training programme.

A 'trainer' is any person other than the tutor who supervises the trainee during part of the preregistration programme. Trainers are usually, but not always, pharmacists. It is the responsibility of the tutor to ensure that trainers have sufficient awareness and understanding of the preregistration programme.

A 'mentor' is someone assigned to the trainee for the duration of the training programme with whom the trainee can have regular meetings to discuss issues of concern. The preregistration tutor is responsible for appointing a suitable mentor to the trainee.

COMPETENCIES

In 1990, preregistration training became competence based with emphasis on vocational training. The training follows a syllabus laid down by the RPSGB and involves achieving and demonstrating a variety of 'competencies'. Competencies are activities considered pivotal to the practice of pharmacy that the student must be able to perform consistently to the required standard (for example, dispensing medicines ordered on a prescription, using a particular piece of apparatus, or counselling patients about the correct use of their medicines). Preregistration tutors are required continually to assess their trainee's competence in performing different tasks. The competencies are described in detail in the *Preregistration Student Manual* and students should expect to work in conjunction with their tutors to ensure compliance with the check lists and the descriptions of competence.

In most placements there will be a specified programme of experience, which may be reinforced by structured training events. It is advisable to enquire about such programmes at interview. Within the training programme regular appraisal reports are completed which should be approved by the student before being forwarded to the Education Division of the RPSGB. A satisfactory 39-week appraisal is a prerequisite for entrance to the registration examination.

THE REGISTRATION EXAMINATION

At the end of the preregistration year, students have to pass a registration examination. The examination was introduced to assess the practice-related knowledge of preregistration trainees and to complement the assessment of their workplace performance.

The London Pharmaceutical Consortium (LPC), comprising The London School of Pharmacy and Edexcel, is responsible for setting the examination questions, drafting the papers, allocating examination centres, and marking the papers. The Education Division of the RPSGB undertakes some of the administrative functions associated with the examination. The examination comprises two two-hour multiple choice question papers. One paper is 'closed book' (100 questions) and the other is 'open book' (70 questions).

The syllabus for the registration examination and the regulations for its conduct are set out in detail in the *Preregistration Student Manual*; both sections are essential reading for all examination candidates.

FURTHER INFORMATION

Royal Pharmaceutical Society of Great Britain. *Code of Practice for Preregistration Recruitment.* London: Royal Pharmaceutical Society of Great Britain, 1997.

Royal Pharmaceutical Society of Great Britain. *Preregistration Student Manual.* London: Royal Pharmaceutical Society of Great Britain, 1997.

Wykes V. The registration examination. *Pharm J* 1997; 259: 853–5.

USEFUL ADDRESSES

British Pharmaceutical Students Association (BPSA)
PO Box 3477
Birmingham B17 8BP

Education Division
Royal Pharmaceutical Society of Great Britain
1 Lambeth High Street
London SE1 7JN

3

Community pharmacy

Community pharmacy is the career choice for 60–65% of pharmacists in Great Britain. Community pharmacists are primarily concerned with the sale and supply of medicines and the provision of advice about medicines, symptoms, and general health matters to the general public.

By law, every community pharmacy in Great Britain should be under the supervision of a pharmacist. The pharmacist must ensure that all legal and ethical requirements are met. *Medicines, Ethics and Practice: A guide for pharmacists*, which is published every six months by the Royal Pharmaceutical Society of Great Britain (RPSGB), assists practising pharmacists to maintain awareness about legislation, the Code of Ethics, professional standards, and general practice issues.

The most important role of the community pharmacist is to dispense medicines ordered on prescription and advise the patient on the correct use of their medicines. Before dispensing any medicine, the pharmacist should check that the dose is appropriate and that the risk of interaction with other medicines that the patient is taking is low. If required, the pharmacist will liaise with the prescriber, ensuring that the patient receives the most appropriate treatment for the presenting condition. This aspect of the pharmacist's role has been facilitated by the introduction of computerised patient medication records in the pharmacy.

Another major role of the community pharmacist is that of responding to symptoms described or presented by members of the public. The pharmacists' knowledge will be used to assess whether the customer should be referred for specialist medical attention or be given an over-the-counter (OTC) medicine. Alternatively, the customer may only require advice or reassurance about their condition.

The community pharmacist is also able to promote awareness on a number of healthcare issues (for example, smoking cessation, contraception, travelling abroad) and many community pharmacies also perform screening tests (for example, blood pressure or cholesterol measurements).

The pharmacist may provide an advisory service about the storage and administration of medicines to the staff of residential homes. The community pharmacist may also be required to visit housebound patients to provide, and advise on the use of, oxygen cylinders and surgical appliances.

Community pharmacists are continually encouraged to maintain and develop their knowledge through attendance at continuing education courses, which may cover various aspects of community practice. In addition, some pharmacists may wish to undertake a further period of study to attain a postgraduate diploma or Masters degree in community pharmacy.

EMPLOYEE COMMUNITY PHARMACIST

The employee community pharmacist can choose whether to work for a large or a small company and select a post that offers the extent of shop management and overall responsibility desired. For example, some employers will require a full management role from the pharmacist, whilst others need a pharmacist to provide only a pharmaceutical service with minimal managerial commitment and paperwork. In the latter case, it would be expected that the employment of staff and the merchandising decisions would be undertaken by the proprietor or company supervisor.

Large companies provide a formal employment environment in order to promote the efficient running of the business. Such a company might offer a structured career progression plan with training provision, pension schemes, and other benefits associated with working for a large company. The pharmacist may choose to change career direction into business management, although this route can result in the pharmaceutical aspects of the job diminishing. Alternatively, those interested in maintaining maximum pharmaceutical involvement may seek career progression to a pharmacy department manager.

Some smaller companies model their business systems on those of their larger competitors, in order to maximise efficiency and profitability, although the working environment may be less formal. The small independent pharmacies are all different, each one reflecting the interests and personality of the owner. Usually less formal, the conditions of employment are varied and often negotiable.

The following points should be considered when applying for an appointment as an employee community pharmacist:

○ what is the total number of hours to be worked each week? It may also be useful to know which days are to be worked and whether you will have lunch breaks (the dispensing of prescriptions and sale of pharmacy medicines must always be supervised by a pharmacist). Is there a possibility of flexibility in the pattern of hours worked each week?

○   what is the basic salary, its review date, and the basis of review? Are there any bonuses and incentives to be aimed for? Are the RPSGB membership fees reimbursed? What payment is made for rota duty or emergency call-outs? Is there any payment for the use of the pharmacist's own transport (for example, for the delivery of oxygen or domiciliary visits)? What provisions are available for sickness, maternity, or childcare leave?

○   what are the opportunities for training and professional development?

○   what are the conditions associated with staff purchases or pricing of stock?

○   is there a contract of employment? If not, insist that a contract be drawn up.

○   is the prospective employer covered by a professional indemnity insurance?

○   is there a pension scheme, contributory or non-contributory?

○   what are the grievance procedures?

○   what is the availability of membership of staff organisations or union membership?

PROPRIETOR PHARMACIST

Usually after a period as an employee, many pharmacists consider becoming a proprietor pharmacist. The achievement of this ambition can be a difficult process but, if successful, practice ownership gives the proprietor pharmacist independence and can be a source of much professional satisfaction.

There are essentially two ways of achieving ownership of a pharmacy: opening a new pharmacy, or purchasing an existing pharmacy business. The further option of franchising a pharmacy from one of the major wholesalers is also discussed below.

Opening a new business

To open a new pharmacy with a National Health Service (NHS) contract (enabling the pharmacy to dispense NHS prescriptions) on a chosen site, an application must be made to the local health authority for consent to provide pharmaceutical services on the site. The application will be considered by the health authority with advice sought from various interested parties including the Local Pharmaceutical Committee (LPC), the Community Health Council (CHC), the Local Medical Committee (LMC), and other pharmacies in the area. The careful selection of a suitable site and good presentation of the case in favour of the proposed pharmacy are vital ingredients if an application is to be successful. Having considered the advice of the interested parties, the health authority may reject the application if it considers the proposed pharmacy to be neither necessary nor desirable. The Secretary of State has delegated responsibility for consideration of appeals against decisions made by local health authority committees to a special appeals unit situated in the Yorkshire region.

If the proposed pharmacy is more than 1 km away from any other pharmacy, it could be eligible for the Essential Small Pharmacies Scheme (ESPS). This scheme can provide a significant subsidy and may make the difference between success and failure.

Permission may need to be sought from the local authority if there is to be a change of use of the premises or if structural alterations are required. The pharmacy must be registered with the RPSGB and careful thought needs to be given towards ensuring compliance with professional requirements regarding the physical layout of the premises. It may be advisable to use the services of specialised shopfitters. The planning department of the National Pharmaceutical Association (NPA) can provide invaluable assistance.

Purchasing an existing business

The capital required to buy an established pharmacy business is likely to be high, perhaps between 25 and 50 pence per pound of annual turnover. This sum, which generally covers the goodwill, fixtures, and fittings must be found in addition to the cost of the stock at valuation. Sometimes the opportunity to purchase the freehold of the premises also arises. This can be an additional financial burden if a mortgage is taken out but may also be an attractive proposition if the premises have suitable living accommodation. Low cost finance packages may be available through the banks, if guaranteed by the major wholesalers. It is important when raising finance to have sound plans and projections to present to the lenders. It is also likely that some personal contribution will be required, perhaps 20% of the total price. Although this may be a daunting prospect, collateral can often be raised from existing assets such as pensions, life assurance, and property. It is wise to seek professional advice at an early stage.

As with opening a new pharmacy, the RPSGB and the local health authority must be contacted. However, arranging formal transfer of the NHS contract is much easier than making a new application. Nevertheless, sufficient time must always be allowed for the formalities to be completed.

The transition from employee to proprietor is an important step. Membership of the NPA is strongly recommended, providing access to advice on professional matters and other services. Additional advice about local conditions should be available from the Local Pharmaceutical Committee (for example, if disputes arise with the health authority or local doctors). The Prescription Pricing Authority, the RPSGB, and its local branch can provide further information and support. Once any initial problems have been successfully solved, life as a proprietor pharmacist can be professionally rewarding and satisfying.

The franchise system

A franchise is defined as 'a commercial concession by which a retailer is granted by a company the generally exclusive right of retailing its goods or providing its services in a specified area, with use of the company's expertise, marketing, trademark, etc.'

This type of system is designed to bring business ownership within the reach of pharmacists who do not possess the capital or collateral to buy or begin a business on their own. The pharmacist can combine the personal service and entrepreneurial skills of a sole trader with the disciplines and support of a multiple.

A franchise may also provide female pharmacists with the opportunity to combine a career and a family, as it may be possible to organise and pay for pharmaceutical cover during the period of maternity leave.

A franchise can be a rewarding venture both professionally and financially but it does require a great deal of commitment. Before taking a franchise it is advisable to discuss the proposal in detail with your bank manager, accountant, and solicitor.

FURTHER INFORMATION

Appelbe GE, Wingfield J. *Dale and Appelbe's Pharmacy Law and Ethics, 6th edition*. London: Pharmaceutical Press, 1997.

Barrow C. *The Complete Small Business Guide, 4th edition*. London: BBC Publications, 1995.

National Pharmaceutical Association. *Matters Requiring Attention Upon Opening a Pharmacy*. St Albans: National Pharmaceutical Association.

National Pharmaceutical Association. *Matters Requiring Attention Upon Buying or Transferring a Business (NPA Notes for Proprietors)*. St Albans: National Pharmaceutical Association.

Royal Pharmaceutical Society of Great Britain. *Medicines, Ethics and Practice: A guide for pharmacists*. London: The Royal Pharmaceutical Society of Great Britain, 1997.

USEFUL ADDRESSES

**British Franchise
Association**
Thames View
Newton Road
Henley-on-Thames
RG9 1HG
Telephone: 01491 578050

**Community Pharmacists
Group**
Royal Pharmaceutical
Society of Great Britain
1 Lambeth High Street
London SE1 7JN
Telephone: 0171 735 9141
(Contact: Miss J Flint)

Moss Chemists
Acquisitions and Franchise
Director
Fern Grove
Feltham
Middlesex TW14 9BD
Telephone: 0181 890 9333
(Contact: Mr M Bayly)

**National Pharmaceutical
Association**
Mallinson House
40–42 St Peter's Street
St Albans
Hertfordshire AL1 3NP
Telephone: 01727 832161

4

Hospital pharmacy

The hospital pharmacy department provides a service for wards and departments within the hospital and also dispenses prescriptions for out-patients. The pharmacy department may also supply some services to members of the healthcare team in the community. The pharmacist offers advice on prescribing, methods of drug use and administration, storage of medicines, and stock levels. Having decided on a career in the hospital sector, pharmacists can choose to work either within the National Health Service (NHS) or within a private hospital environment.

WARD AND CLINICAL PHARMACY

Pharmacists have a detailed knowledge of clinical pharmacology, therapeutics, pharmaceutics, and pharmaceutical chemistry. The application of this knowledge within the hospital environment enables the pharmacist to assist with prescribing decisions, suggest alternative treatments where necessary, identify instances where the medication administered to a patient for one condition is exacerbating another condition, and to identify an adverse reaction caused by excipients or additives within a formulation.

On a ward visit, the pharmacist examines the prescription sheet for newly prescribed items. The pharmacist also checks other charts such as intravenous therapy, diabetic monitoring, or anticoagulant therapy. New patients are asked about previous drug therapy to identify possible problems. The ward stocks are checked and any additional items are ordered. The pharmacist promotes compliance with local prescribing policies and promotes the economical use of drugs and nursing items.

Clinical pharmacists are encouraged to take part in drug and therapeutics committees within hospitals where there is an opportunity to promote cost-effective prescribing and rationalise drug usage. Attendance at consultant ward rounds is often requested. Clinical pharmacists may also be involved with out-patient clinics, for example, anticoagulant clinics. Pharmacists are often encouraged to study for a diploma or Masters degree in clinical pharmacy.

DRUG INFORMATION

The provision of information on drugs is traditionally part of the role of every pharmacist, but in recent years several factors have influenced and stimulated the development of drug information as a speciality. The number of new medicines, many with increased potency and selectivity, has risen markedly. This has been paralleled by a dramatic growth in the volume and complexity of biomedical literature.

The rising cost of new treatments, at a time of financial constraints within the NHS, together with intense commercial promotion and the expansion of hospital pharmacy services into ward and clinical activities have all contributed to the need for specialist drug information services within hospital pharmacy departments. Although drug information has developed as a specialised function of the hospital pharmaceutical service, it serves both the hospital and community healthcare sectors.

The aim of the drug information service is to promote the safe, effective, and economic use of medicinal products in patients by the active and passive provision of drug information and advice. This is achieved through a network of drug information centres throughout the country. Nearly every local unit now has a designated pharmacist who is responsible for drug information. Most centres are supported by a regional centre.

A large proportion of a drug information pharmacist's time is spent answering enquiries. Enquiries can cover all aspects of drug use, although enquiries about poisoning are usually referred to poisons information centres. Enquiries about the adverse effects of drugs constitute an ever-increasing part of drug information work. In view of this, adverse drug reaction monitoring programmes have been developed in some centres.

Pharmacists may be asked to identify unfamiliar drugs (perhaps foreign products or clinical trial supplies) and to establish a supply route or to suggest an alternative. Enquiries about drug interactions and interactions between drugs and food or drugs and laboratory tests are also frequently received.

A variety of sources are available to the pharmacist when answering an enquiry. These include a range of textbooks, journals, manufacturers' literature, in-house databases, and commercial computerised databases either via on-line or CD-ROM facilities. External sources such as the Information Centre at the Royal Pharmaceutical Society of Great Britain, medical information departments within the pharmaceutical industry, and many groups (including self-help groups with specialist knowledge) are invaluable to the information pharmacist.

The production of regular bulletins for various groups of staff also features prominently in the workload. Increasingly, drug information pharmacists are becoming involved in supporting local drug and therapeutics committees.

Hospital drug information centres are also becoming increasingly involved with the provision of a service to the community sector. Support is often provided to medical and pharmaceutical advisers and assistance is offered with the promulgation and production of practice and health authority formularies. The growing importance of the primary care sector means that this drug information role will continue to develop in the future.

PHARMACEUTICAL PRODUCTION

Pharmaceutical production departments in hospitals have two main functions: bulk manufacture of pharmaceuticals and specialised dispensing (on a named-patient basis).

Manufacturing processes in hospitals must comply with regulations specified in the Medicines Act 1968. In addition, manufacturing units must have an appropriate licence from the Medicines Control Agency (MCA). Compliance with the *Rules and Guidance for Pharmaceutical Manufacturers, The Rules Governing Medicinal Products in the European Community, Volume IV* and European Community Directives on Good Manufacturing Practice (GMP) is vital. Manufacturing units must also comply with health and safety legislation.

The most common manufacturing activity within hospitals is the repackaging of medicines. Sterile dispensing is another major function of the pharmaceutical production department. It is defined as the preparation of any sterile medicine for an individual named patient (for example, parenteral nutrition, cytotoxic preparations, or a central intravenous additive service (CIVAS)). Radiopharmaceuticals may also be prepared. The manufacturing department within a hospital may also offer a service producing 'specials' (unlicensed preparations for individual patients). The considerable investment required to establish and maintain a pharmaceutical production unit has resulted in the closure of many hospital units. Of the few units that remain, most offer a centralised service.

QUALITY ASSURANCE

The quality assurance laboratory within a pharmacy department must ensure that products are consistently of a quality appropriate to their intended use. Compliance with this remit requires strict operating procedures, modern and well-maintained equipment, and dedicated staff.

The quality assurance department must monitor:

○ goods manufactured in the pharmaceutical production unit;

○ medicines dispensed in the dispensary;

○ storage and distribution procedures;

○ medical gas supplies;

○ accuracy of quality control.

NATIONAL HEALTH SERVICE – HOSPITAL TRUSTS

Most hospitals in Great Britain are now managed as independent business units with a board consisting of five executive and five non-executive directors, with a chairman who is appointed by the Secretary of State for Health. Trust hospitals are now outside the regional structure and are directly responsible to the Minister of Health.

In the pharmacy department, pharmacists will be employed with technicians and other support staff. The pharmacist is now considered to be part of the hospital support team working with doctors and nurses to provide the best service for the patient.

Career progression and training

Pharmacists who have little experience of hospital practice are usually appointed to a training grade (A or B) to gain experience in most aspects of the department before moving on to specialise or to obtain managerial expertise running a section such as out-patient services.

Most pharmacists participate in a performance review process, which involves agreeing job objectives and a personal development plan. This plan identifies development and training needs to help career progression. There may be opportunities to study for diplomas or higher degrees in clinical pharmacy.

Flexible working

Most hospital pharmacists work full-time and many combine a successful career with raising a family. There are often opportunities for part-time work and job-sharing. Flexi-time and workplace nurseries may also be available.

Career breaks

National Health Service employees are able to take career breaks of up to five years to start a family or to care for elderly or disabled relatives. The agreement between NHS management and unions covers both men and women and allows local managers flexibility on how the scheme is implemented. The leave is unpaid except for a work requirement of ten days per year. There is no guarantee of the same job on returning to work, but similar duties and pay should apply. Pharmacy managers are aware of the needs of those who have had a career break. They should be able to organise a familiarisation programme enabling the 'returner' to join the pharmacy team.

A planned programme enables the returning pharmacist to learn about the duties of clinical pharmacists on the ward and to experience the clinical team approach with doctors and nurses. As experience is gained, the pharmacist may choose to specialise in one of the departments within the hospital pharmacy or, alternatively, the pharmacist may wish to work within the community services sector (*see also* Chapter 8).

Those considering a return to work (whether full-time or part-time, flexible hours, or job-share) are advised to contact the chief pharmacist or director of pharmaceutical services at the local hospital. A visit to the hospital pharmacy is recommended to discuss employment opportunities in person and to meet the staff.

The chief pharmacist will be able to provide up-to-date information on salaries. There is a nationally agreed salary structure but trusts are able to negotiate salaries locally, which may not coincide with nationally recommended scales and are therefore not subject to the Whitley Council Scales.

Some hospital pharmacies hold a list of bank pharmacists available for part-time work and will give some update training.

Further information about this subject is given in Chapter 10.

PRIVATE HOSPITAL SECTOR

The number of independent acute hospitals in Great Britain is growing rapidly. Hospital sizes vary from about 30–300 beds. There are opportunities for full-time, part-time, job-share, and locum pharmacists. When recruiting staff, pharmacists with hospital experience are preferred and the ability to work in a multidisciplinary team is essential.

Managing the pharmaceutical service in a private hospital entails controlling the budget, organising the supply and storage of all pharmaceuticals in the hospital, dispensing for in-patients (and possibly out-patients), and providing a 24-hour drug information and advice service.

Those interested in working in a private hospital should contact the secretary of the Association of Private Hospital Pharmacists (APHP), who will provide details of the hospitals in a specified area. The Association of Private Hospital Pharmacists organises study meetings, lectures, and discussions on topical issues. In addition, it arranges social gatherings, providing members with the opportunity to meet and discuss common issues. The association has published guidelines on the minimum standards for pharmaceutical services in independent acute hospitals.

FURTHER INFORMATION

Commission of the European Communities. *The Rules Governing Medicinal Products in the European Community, Volume IV: Good Manufacturing Practice for Medicinal Products*. Luxembourg: Commission of the European Communities, 1995.

Medicines Control Agency. *Rules and Guidance for Pharmaceutical Manufacturers*. London: HMSO, 1993.

Stone P, Curtis SJ. *Pharmacy Practice, 2nd edition*. London: Farrand Press, 1995.

The Hospital Pharmacy (video produced by Bristol Myers Squibb)
Audio Visual Services
Royal Pharmaceutical Society of Great Britain
1 Lambeth High Street
London SE1 7JN
Telephone: 0171 735 9141 Ext 288 (ref PRA8)

USEFUL ADDRESSES

Association of Private
Hospital Pharmacists
Hospital of St John and
St Elizabeth
60 Grove End Road
London NW8 9NH
Telephone: 0171 286 5126
Ext 337
(Contact: Mrs J Baxter)

College of Pharmacy
Practice
University of Warwick
Science Park
Barclays Venture Centre
Coventry
West Midlands
CV4 7EZ
Telephone: 01203 692400

**Drug Information
Pharmacists Group**
Trent Drug Information
Centre
Leicester Royal Infirmary
Leicester LE1 5WW
Telephone: 0116 255 5779
(Contact: Mr P Golightly)

**Guild of Hospital
Pharmacists**
50 Southwark Street
London SE1 1UN
Telephone: 0171 717 4000

**Hospital Pharmacists
Group**
Royal Pharmaceutical
Society of Great Britain
1 Lambeth High Street
London SE1 7JN
Telephone: 0171 735 9141

**National Association
of Senior Pharmacy
Managers and
Advisers**
Pharmacy Department
Wexham Park Hospital
Slough
Berkshire SL2 4HL
Telephone: 01753 633000
Ext 3100
(Contact: Mr RH Higson)

**United Kingdom Clinical
Pharmacy Association**
Alpha House
Countesthorpe Road
South Wigston
Leicestershire
LE18 4PJ
Telephone: 01162 776999
(Contact: Mrs S Shaw)

5

Industrial pharmacy

The opportunities for pharmacists in industrial pharmacy, whether in the pharmaceutical industry or in the cosmetics industry, are as varied as the companies themselves. The 300 or so companies that make up the industry in Great Britain share a common need for pharmacists who are able to play key roles in many different areas. The companies vary greatly in size and complexity – from research-based multi-nationals through contract and generic companies to single-product operations. Pharmacists account for approximately 1.5% of the workforce in the industry.

PHARMACEUTICAL INDUSTRY

Many new graduates entering the pharmaceutical industry opt for a post where the pharmacist's skills are of direct and unquestioned value, such as development, quality assurance, or production. Later, having gained some experience and knowledge of the industry, they can decide whether to develop more specialist professional skills or seek a move into another area such as registration or marketing.

Research

Pharmaceutical research involves the discovery or design of novel, biologically active molecules in a therapeutically useful form. The research and development process for a new chemical entity may occupy six to twelve years and demand an investment of some £150 million.

The composition of the research team varies, but typically includes medicinal chemists, pharmacologists, biochemists, microbiologists, analytical chemists, toxicologists, and statisticians. Pharmacists who wish to enter basic research must specialise and undertake further study in one of the relevant fields. Although this may be done by research for a higher degree, most companies are willing to give on-the-job training to scientists who can demonstrate an ability to learn and contribute in specialist fields.

Apart from the more specialised roles, research laboratories also require co-ordinators to assist in the scheduling of research and the documentation and dissemination of results. More recently, the introduction of international 'good laboratory practice' standards has created additional roles for assuring the integrity and quality of safety and toxicity studies.

Development

During the development stage, the potency, purity, stability, and bioavailability of the active substance is investigated, leading to the preparation of the final formulation. Once the formulation has been developed, clinical trials are carried out to assess the efficacy, safety, and toxicity of the preparation. Towards the end of the development stage, pilot plant studies are necessary to confirm that both the active substance and the final formulation can be manufactured on an industrial scale.

Each development activity requires constant liaison between many disciplines if the prime objective of getting the best product to the market in the shortest time is to be achieved. The broad training of pharmacists equips them well for this interface. Additionally, the pharmaceutics and clinical pharmacy contents of the undergraduate course make pharmacy an appropriate discipline for product formulation and related activities.

Clinical trials

Assessing the effectiveness of a new drug or of a new presentation of an established one is an essential part of the development of a medicine. Trials in humans normally involve four phases: assessment in healthy human volunteers, controlled clinical trials in small numbers of patients, large scale safety and efficacy studies, and controlled post-marketing studies in patients.

The preparation and presentation of clinical trial materials must comply with study protocols. Packaging, labelling, and distribution must all be performed to established 'good manufacturing practice' and 'good clinical practice' standards and must satisfy all regulatory requirements.

Opportunities for pharmacists include involvement in the manufacture and supply of clinical trial materials. In addition, the pharmacist is ideally qualified to be a clinical research associate involved in the planning, monitoring, and reporting of clinical trials. The role involves liaison with scientists and clinicians at all levels within the company and at clinical trial sites. It also involves frequent visits to study centres, which could provide the opportunity for foreign travel.

Production

Production is central to the growth and success of a pharmaceutical organisation, and the quality and efficiency of manufacturing systems are key elements in the strategy of any healthcare corporation. Manufacturing processes may be concerned with the production of the drug substance itself (bulk or primary production) or with the production of medicinal products (pharmaceutical or secondary production). It is the latter area which attracts the majority of production pharmacists. Pharmaceutical production is further divided according to dosage forms (solid, liquid, and sterile products).

The efficient management of materials is important and computer-based techniques are generally used for controlling stocks. The design and application of computer-based systems are likely to be important elements in the production pharmacist's job description.

The production pharmacist carries responsibility for the use of equipment that varies in complexity from a simple bench-mounted unit to a fully automated packaging or manufacturing line. Involvement in solving day-to-day problems arising from equipment and material malfunction is an integral part of the job. There is also a role for the pharmacist in the development and modification of pharmaceutical processes. Production departments usually employ relatively large numbers of people; therefore, the production pharmacist should possess good leadership and management skills.

Quality management

Examination of all aspects that contribute to the quality of a finished pharmaceutical product requires wide knowledge and experience covering everything from original design, development and formulation through various manufacturing and packaging stages to the decision point where the product is released into the distribution chain.

Within the European Community, legislation also demands that the release of fully licensed medicinal products onto the market is undertaken by a 'qualified person'. The pharmacy undergraduate course provides much of the theoretical knowledge required for registration as a qualified person.

Quality management can include the following activities:

○ procurement of raw materials and packaging components and the subsequent control of these in the factory;

○ consideration of the design of premises and environmental requirements;

○ process and analytical development including stability and shelf-life determination;

○ design and implementation of pharmaceutical quality systems including documentation and standard operating procedures;

○ application of computers to improve information and data handling relating to material and product release;

○ validation of pharmaceutical utilities, equipment, and processes;

○ training of personnel in quality assurance, manufacturing, engineering, and warehousing;

○ auditing and self-inspection to ensure maintenance of standards and compliance with regulation;

○ liaison with company regulatory departments to ensure compliance with licensing commitments;

○   general factory organisation and the procedures adopted to enable compliance with good pharmaceutical manufacturing practice;

○   sound technical and professional knowledge of company products covering not only their action and use, but also a practical understanding of manufacturing and packaging processes for major dosage forms;

○   quality control laboratory management of the many procedures that constitute good control laboratory practice.

Pharmacists in quality management, especially those working as qualified persons, work closely with many other specialist disciplines, enabling them to use their background knowledge to understand and contribute to the many facets of manufacture and control that help to assure the quality of the finished product. The pharmacist working in quality management must also have a thorough knowledge of current national and international pharmaceutical legislation.

Marketing

Marketing is one of the most important components in the development of a new medicine. Marketing personnel must be knowledgeable about the clinical profile of the product, the economics of development and production, and the techniques of marketing and selling. Involvement in the development of a new product entails estimating customer needs and also participating in the preparation of target profiles for research planning. In addition, the marketing department must forecast the long-term commercial demand and therefore determine how the production process will be planned.

Members of marketing departments may also determine possible improvements to, or additional uses for, existing drugs by studying clinical reports.

A company may appoint a product manager to be responsible for the marketing and subsequent profitability of a product. The product manager must identify the key features of a product that should be emphasised in the promotion campaign. The responsibility for bringing these features to the attention of doctors and pharmacists rests partly with the company's team of field-based medical representatives. Composition of mailing shots and journal advertisements are also the responsibility of the product manager.

Pharmacists are also well qualified to fulfil the role of a medical representative. Representatives must communicate effectively with healthcare professionals and pharmacists have the technical and professional background that enables them to achieve this. Further marketing opportunities for pharmacists include market research and training roles.

Regulatory affairs

The requirements of regulatory authorities throughout the world are comprehensive and very complex. Most of the activities of pharmaceutical companies are regulated to varying degrees – from research and development stages through to sales and marketing. In an increasing number of cases, there is an additional requirement for specific post-marketing monitoring of a new medicine. The objective of these regulations is to ensure the quality, safety, and efficacy of medicinal products.

When a new drug substance enters development, quality has to be adequately determined for both the drug substance and the final formulation. The stability of the formulation must also be assessed to determine a shelf-life. Before an application is made for an authorisation to market, full-scale manufacturing processes have to be developed and validated. A programme of toxicology studies must be designed to meet international requirements and these must be performed in accordance with 'good laboratory practice' standards. Clinical trials must be performed to assess safety and efficacy in humans and these must be conducted in accordance with 'good clinical practice' standards. Approval from the regulatory authorities may be required to conduct these clinical studies. Teamwork is essential in this process, as any delay in obtaining regulatory clearance for new products can be extremely costly to the company.

Approvals to conduct clinical trials are required in many countries. The format and content of the application varies; some countries require only summaries of the available data, whereas others require that all supporting data is submitted. These approvals need continuous updating as trials are completed and new studies are proposed.

The marketing authorisation application contains the results of all the work carried out during development and is usually presented in three sections – the chemistry and pharmacy data (which supports the quality of the product), the preclinical pharmacology and toxicology studies (which provide evidence of safety), and the clinical studies (which provide evidence of efficacy and safety in humans). It is the role of regulatory affairs personnel to submit the application and also to negotiate with the authorities to gain regulatory approval for the product. Marketing authorisations must also be renewed at regular intervals, involving the preparation of further documentation by regulatory personnel.

The regulatory affairs department is involved with many other activities relating to successful commercialisation of new and existing products. This would include liaison with colleagues about the generation of all forms of product literature including labels, package inserts, summaries of product characteristics, information leaflets, and promotional materials. After the launch of new products, there is a requirement for specific reporting of adverse events to the regulatory authorities – a procedure known as post-marketing surveillance. There is an ongoing need to notify the authorities about changes to the original data; for example, if manufacturing or quality control procedures are modified, or if new clinical data become available that support a new therapeutic use for a product. Each alteration to the original application requires the submission of an application for a variation to the licence, along with justification for the change.

In addition, the regulatory affairs department is responsible for the renewal of manufacturers and wholesale dealers' licences. Regulatory personnel have a responsibility to keep abreast with all changes in regulatory directives and guidelines, both national and international. Career prospects for regulatory affairs personnel are excellent. Following the opening of the European Medicines Evaluation Agency in London in 1995, major changes in product registration are taking place. Product registration is recognised as pivotal to the success of a pharmaceutical company.

Information

The role of the information scientist involves co-ordination and contact with a range of disciplines, both inside and outside the company. Within the pharmaceutical industry departments specialise in both medical and scientific information.

Medical

Information about a company's product comes from a range of sources – international literature, adverse reaction and drug interaction reports, special communications, and clinical research. Each piece of information must be evaluated for scientific significance and then indexed so that it may be retrieved when necessary; such activities build a product database. In most medical information units the database is computerised, leading to involvement with electronic data processing staff and the opportunity for hands-on experience of new technology and the use of external databases. The experience gained by information personnel when assessing and indexing information gives them detailed and specialised knowledge of the company's products, the relevant therapeutic groups, and the diseases for which they may be used.

A major part of the information scientist's role is to respond to enquiries from healthcare professionals and also the general public. The information department also provides technical support to other departments within the company, such as those dealing with marketing, regulatory affairs, and clinical research.

The information pharmacist may be involved with the following:

○ writing data sheets;
○ writing technical booklets;
○ approving advertising copy;
○ writing label text and patient leaflets;

○ advising marketing staff;

○ training medical representatives;

○ pharmacovigilance, adverse drug reaction monitoring;

○ organising a medical library.

Scientific

Pharmacists in this discipline are usually based in the research and development division and provide current awareness, retrospective, and on-line searching of the scientific and medical literature, and maintain document archives. Scientific information scientists may also provide information on competitor products. This field can provide the pharmacist with the opportunity to combine interests in literature and research.

COSMETICS INDUSTRY

Opportunities for pharmacists also exist in the cosmetics industry, dealing with skin care, toiletries, and decorative cosmetics. Although a degree in pharmacy may not be essential for the majority of opportunities in the cosmetics industry, pharmacists are eminently qualified to work in a variety of departments, such as research and development, production, quality control, post-marketing surveillance, marketing, or sales. Work within each department is similar to that in the pharmaceutical industry. However, as there are fewer regulatory constraints, the cosmetics industry has more scope to produce innovative formulations and bring these to market more quickly. Jobs in the cosmetics industry are unlikely to be advertised in the pharmaceutical press; companies should be contacted directly to discuss opportunities for employment.

USEFUL ADDRESSES

Association of Information Officers in the Pharmaceutical Industry (AIOPI)
Medical Information Department
Bristol Myers Squibb
141–149 Staines Road
Hounslow
Middlesex TW3 3JB
Telephone: 0181 570 1888
(Contact: Ms G Eastby)

Association of the British Pharmaceutical Industry (ABPI)
12 Whitehall
London SW1A 2DY
Telephone: 0171 930 3477

British Institute of Regulatory Affairs
Ground Floor
7 Heron Quays
London E14 4JB
Telephone: 0171 538 9502

Cosmetic Toiletry & Perfumery Association Ltd
Josaron House
5–7 John Princes Street
London W1M 9HD
Telephone: 0171 491 8891

Industrial Pharmacists Group
Royal Pharmaceutical
Society of Great Britain
1 Lambeth High Street
London SE1 7JN
Telephone: 0171 735 9141
(Contact: Miss J Flint)

Institute of Quality Assurance
54 Princess Gate
Exhibition Road
London
SW7 2PG
Telephone: 0171 584 9026

Pharmaceutical Marketing Society
PO Box 200
Horsham
West Sussex RH13 3FA
Telephone: 01403 264898
(Contact: Ms V Bennett)

Pharmaceutical Quality Group
c/o Organon Ltd
New House
Motherwell
Lanarkshire ML1 5SH
Telephone: 01698 732611
(Contact: Mr I Richardson)

Society of Cosmetic Scientists
GT House
24–26 Rothesay Road
Luton
Bedfordshire LU1 1QX
Telephone: 01582 26661

6

Education

A career in education can be both rewarding and fulfilling. It can also provide the pharmacist interested in research with the opportunity to further their postgraduate studies, possibly leading to the attainment of a higher degree.

SCHOOLS OF PHARMACY

In the past, the path to a career in academia required the attainment of a first or upper second class honours degree in pharmacy, followed by completion of the preregistration year, before obtaining a Doctor of Philosophy degree (PhD). Today, recruitment in schools of pharmacy involves the assessment of academic and other appropriate qualifications and experience.

Each pharmacy school produces a research prospectus, copies of which can be obtained by contacting the schools directly. Specific research positions are normally advertised in *The Pharmaceutical Journal* or other relevant publications. The research involved may lead to a higher degree (MPhil or PhD) or may be postdoctoral.

A variety of different types of employment contract is available in this sector of the profession, including full-time academic, part-time academic, job-share academic, or teacher-practitioner (*see* below). The precise details of the contract will vary depending on the school of pharmacy, the teaching area, and the level (undergraduate or postgraduate), but the work may include the following:

○   design, implementation, and evaluation of lectures, course-work assignments, practicals (pharmacy practice or laboratory based), workshops, tutorials, projects, and assessments;

○   assessment of knowledge, skills, and competence;

○   research leading to publications;

○   study or research for additional qualifications;

○   acting as personal tutor to students;

○   attending meetings within department, faculty, university, or off-site;

○   liaison with other organisations with an interest in pharmacy.

THE TEACHER-PRACTITIONER

A teacher-practitioner pharmacist is employed to work in practice, undertake research, and teach; each component is carried out to a significant, but variable, extent. The teacher-practitioner works at the interface of practice and academia. Moreover, the emergence of practitioners with a contractual commitment to a school of pharmacy has facilitated the influence of practice on academic direction. Teacher-practitioner posts have also encouraged the development of practice research. However, perhaps the most important effect of the teacher-practitioner role has been to improve the degree of contact between the pharmacy student and the patient. This contact helps the student relate science to practice and promotes the understanding of the problems faced by the patient.

The individual may practice in the hospital, community, or industrial sector. The majority of teacher-practitioners tend to work in hospitals; however, the introduction of sponsored placements of community-based teacher-practitioners into most schools of pharmacy has redressed the balance to some extent. At present, there are few teacher-practitioners working in the pharmaceutical industry.

Job descriptions for teacher-practitioner posts vary greatly. Some teacher-practitioners are employed to work 90% of their time in the practice environment with the remaining time allocated to teaching. For others, the time commitments may be the exact opposite. The ideal division of time has been considered to be in the order of a 50:50 or 75:25 (practice:academic) split, depending on the nature of the individual's responsibilities.

The principal subjects taught by teacher-practitioners vary, although they are usually closely related to the individual's practice and research activities. The most common subjects taught by teacher-practitioners are pharmacokinetics, therapeutics, and pharmacy practice. The teaching can be at the undergraduate, postgraduate, or in-service level. Pharmacists interested in becoming teacher-practitioners must be enthusiastic about practice and academia, and should be willing to follow an alternative career structure.

TECHNICAL COLLEGES

The training of pharmacy technicians in technical colleges (tertiary colleges) provides another teaching opportunity for the pharmacist. Possession of a higher degree or qualification in education is not essential. These training positions may not be advertised; therefore, interested parties are advised to contact the head of department at the appropriate college.

SECONDARY SCHOOLS

A shortfall in the number of science teachers in secondary education is anticipated; providing opportunities for science graduates in all disciplines, including pharmacy. In order to qualify as a secondary school teacher, one must normally attain a Postgraduate Certificate of Education (PGCE). Although a pharmacy graduate may be eligible to apply for the post of a science teacher without further qualifications being necessary, the Department for Education and Employment recommends that a training course is undertaken in order to gain experience and develop confidence in conveying a subject to others.

The entrance to a PGCE course should be straightforward for a pharmacy graduate wishing to change career direction, providing the pharmacy degree course included two years of chemistry. A grant may be available from the local authority and a bursary may also be available. The course is full-time, half of which is spent on teaching practice; a number of PGCE courses offer a distance learning package. Once the further qualification has been achieved, there are opportunities to become a secondary school teacher or an Open University tutor, to teach at adult education classes, or to tutor children privately for examinations. External moderators are also required for General Certificate of Secondary Education (GCSE) assessments.

USEFUL ADDRESSES

**Centre for Pharmacy
Postgraduate Education**
School of Pharmacy and
Pharmaceutical Sciences
University of Manchester
Oxford Road
Manchester
M13 9PL
Telephone: 0161 275 2324

Open University
PO Box 48
Milton Keynes MK7 6AB

**TASC (Teaching as a
Career) Unit**
35 Great Smith Street
London SW1P 3BW
Telephone: 0171 222 8100

7

Locum pharmacy

Opportunities for locum work exist in all branches of the profession. However, the majority of opportunities for locum pharmacists are in the community sector. A prospective locum should assess the demand for locum work in the selected geographical area and advertise their availability for such work. In practical terms, this can mean visits to local pharmacies, telephone calls to local hospitals, inclusion in the Royal Pharmaceutical Society of Great Britain branch locum lists, and registering with a locum agency. Information about standard locum fees can be found in advertisements in the pharmaceutical press and by talking to other locums.

PERSONAL COMMUNICATION WITH EMPLOYERS

When dealing directly with a prospective employer, the locum should check all the arrangements and negotiate to resolve any problems. Relevant details will include the venue, dates and times of employment, whether or not there is a lunch break, whether travelling expenses are paid, and discussion about any special features or requirements of the pharmacy. The locum should establish payment procedures and also whether substitutes may be sent. All terms and conditions should be agreed before starting work, and it is good practice to confirm them in writing as this protects both parties and avoids misunderstandings that could prove to be expensive.

LOCUM AGENCIES

The alternative to direct communication with employers is to register with a reputable locum agency. The agency deals with all arrangements and practical details on behalf of the locum, who simply has to decide where and when to work and for how long.

Agencies are playing an increasingly important role in establishing nationally accepted terms, rates, and conditions for locums. On an annual basis, they are involved in reviews of locum rates with employers. The agency may also organise locum training courses, produce locum magazines, assist in resolving disputes between locums and employers, or provide support to locums when dealing with the Inland Revenue.

TAXATION

Self-employed locums have an advantage over their colleagues who are employed by a single employer with regard to income tax. In the past, the Inland Revenue did attempt to operate a pay-as-you-earn system for all locums. However, after a national campaign, it was agreed that locum pharmacists would continue to be treated as self-employed individuals provided that they strictly adhere to the pertinent rules.

INSURANCE

The *Code of Ethics and Professional Standards* (incorporated within *Medicines, Ethics and Practice: A guide for pharmacists*, which is published every six months by the Royal

Pharmaceutical Society of Great Britain) states that all pharmacists must work with the full protection of professional indemnity insurance. A locum should check that they are covered by indemnity insurance at every pharmacy in which they work. Alternatively, pharmacists can take out personal indemnity insurance, which provides protection irrespective of whether the pharmacy is covered.

Even when working in a pharmacy whose professional indemnity insurance covers the activities of the locum, situations can arise where a proprietor takes action against the locum. The proprietor's professional indemnity insurance will not protect the locum in this situation. Locums are therefore strongly advised to look carefully at their professional indemnity insurance arrangements. At the very least, they should have personal insurance cover for legal defence costs.

FURTHER INFORMATION

Benefits Agency. *Self-Employed? Booklet FB30.* Leeds: Benefits Agency.

Mason P. *Locum Pharmacy: A survival guide.* London: Pharmaceutical Press, 1998.

USEFUL ADDRESSES

Benefits Agency
Quarry House
Quarry Hill
Leeds LS2 7UA
Telephone: 0113 232 4000

8

Pharmaceutical advisers and community services pharmacists

Reforms to the National Health Service (NHS) in the 1980s brought new roles and responsibilities for pharmacists. Further information on these reforms can be found in relevant publications including *Working for Patients* (and its derivatives), *Promoting Better Health*, and *Improving Prescribing*.

THE PHARMACEUTICAL ADVISER

Following the creation of the NHS in 1948, there were few restraints on prescribing practice. However, concern about the increasing NHS drugs bill prompted the introduction of the Limited List in 1985 (now called the Selected List Scheme). This initial measure was followed by further NHS reforms concerned with lowering prescribing costs.

In 1989, the document *Working for Patients* set out the General Practitioner Fundholding Scheme and the Indicative Prescribing Scheme for non-fundholding general practitioners where each general practice is set an indicative amount for prescribing costs, which should not be exceeded during the financial year. This indicative amount or Target Budget is the estimated amount of money each general practitioner practice will spend on prescribing during the year. The aim was to focus attention on drug use and prescribing costs.

Other recommendations on general practitioner prescribing, highlighted in *Improving Prescribing*, included improving the access that general practitioners have to prescribing data through prescribing analyses and cost tables (PACT), encouraging the development of practice formularies, and providing medical and pharmaceutical advice for general practitioners by doctors and pharmacists based in health authorities.

Health authorities administer contracts for independent contractors (doctors, dentists, pharmacists, and opticians), and now have the responsibilities for implementing many of the primary care reforms such as the Indicative Prescribing Scheme. In the publication *Improving Prescribing*, it was stated that 'general practitioners will be provided with information and educational support to examine critically prescribing patterns and costs.' Medical and pharmaceutical adviser posts were, therefore, created to encourage doctors to improve their prescribing.

The pharmaceutical adviser's main task is to promote the rational and cost-effective use of medicines within the primary healthcare services. The pharmaceutical adviser works closely with the medical adviser (where the post exists) who is responsible for general practitioner prescribing and the broader issues of general practice.

Most of the pharmaceutical adviser's time is spent on prescribing issues, which may involve visits to general practitioners to discuss their prescribing patterns. The pharmaceutical adviser acts as a source of independent advice on drug treatment, analyses and interprets PACT data, and assists general practitioners with the development of practice-based formularies.

Many pharmaceutical advisers have a background in hospital drug information work and may produce written advice on drug costs and usage, in addition to answering enquiries by telephone and during practice visits. Enquiries from general practitioners cover a wide range of issues; for example, service fees for the administration of vaccines, arrangements for drug treatment for a patient going abroad, or whether a product is reimbursable on prescription form FP10.

Other responsibilities include liaison with hospital and community pharmacists on prescribing issues and monitoring aspects of the pharmacy contractors' contract such as services to residential homes, practice leaflets, and patient medication records.

Liaison with hospital pharmacists involves occasional meetings with pharmacy managers to discuss specific issues, such as shared-care arrangements. The cost-shifting of expensive drugs by hospitals into the community (for example, if a consultant prescribes a preparation initially but then asks the general practitioner to continue long-term prescribing) may require consultation with medical and pharmaceutical advisers.

Advisers also attend hospital drug and therapeutics committees where many of these issues are discussed. Hospital decisions about drug treatment and the choice of drugs stocked by the pharmacy are likely to have an impact on general practitioner prescribing costs in the community. High volume, lower cost drugs such as diuretics, which hospitals buy as loss leaders (drugs which cost considerably less in hospital compared to community practice) is also a major area of discussion.

Liaison with community pharmacists may involve the development of a strategy for community pharmaceutical services, setting standards and targets, monitoring aspects of the contract and attending local pharmaceutical committee meetings. Health authorities now have schemes for the collection and disposal of unwanted medicines by community pharmacies and these may be administered by the pharmaceutical adviser.

Pharmaceutical advisers have formed a national group with a representative from each NHS region. A survey by the group in 1993 found that the majority of pharmaceutical adviser posts were part-time, with responsibility often shared between the health authority and a hospital post. Job descriptions vary but prescribing issues are usually a priority. Several major reports, for example, that of the House of Commons Select Committee on the National Health Service (July 1994) have recommended that pharmaceutical advisers should be appointed to all health authorities.

THE COMMUNITY SERVICES PHARMACIST

A considerable amount of healthcare is provided through community clinics managed and funded by health authorities and NHS trusts Many clinics are staffed by community nurses, health visitors, and various therapists and chiropodists. Some also have doctors and dentists in attendance at certain times. Many units now have pharmacists or senior technicians with responsibility for providing a pharmaceutical service to community clinics. They visit the clinics on a regular basis to assess the needs of the establishment and the best methods of supply. The range of items used in clinics is vast; there is, therefore, a need for pharmaceutical advice and support.

There is much variety in the way in which community services pharmacists undertake their work. Following the introduction of the 'purchaser/provider' split within the NHS and the creation of hospital trusts, some community services pharmacists are 'providers', and others are 'purchasers'.

The provider role involves:

○ supply of vaccines and pharmaceuticals to clinics and general practitioners;

○ provision of advice and training of community healthcare staff;

○ involvement with discharge planning, including liaison with community pharmacists, social services, and other members of the multi-disciplinary team;

○ involvement in relocation programmes for patients from long stay hospitals being resettled in the community;

○ advice on public health issues such as drug abuse and family planning.

The purchaser role involves:

○ membership of the health authority registration team for the registration and inspection of nursing homes;

○ provision of advice to social services inspection teams, regarding use of medicines in residential homes and training of care staff;

○ some public health issues such as co-ordination of needle and syringe exchange schemes.

The variety of roles undertaken by community services pharmacists ensures that they have practical knowledge and understanding of local health and social care networks.

The Community Services Pharmacists Group was formed in 1986.

USEFUL ADDRESSES

Community Services
Pharmacists Group
Inspection Officer
Pharmacist
East Norfolk Health
Authority
St Andrews Business Park
Thorpe St Andrew
Norwich
Norfolk
NR7 0HT
Telephone: 01603 300600
Ext 313
(Contact: Ms H
Sommerville)

Pharmaceutical Advisers
Group
103 Manor Road
Wallasey
Merseyside M45 7LU
(Contact: Ms C Dutton)

Pharmaceutical and Medical
Advisers Forum (Wales)
Bro Taf Health Authority
Churchill House
Churchill Way
Cardiff CF1 4TW
Telephone: 01222 374731
(Contact: Dr B Davies)

9

Further career options

In addition to the career paths discussed so far, pharmacists can also find rewarding opportunities in areas as varied as veterinary science, the Civil Service, medical journalism and the Prison Pharmaceutical Service.

AGRICULTURAL AND VETERINARY PHARMACY

There are a number of career opportunities for pharmacists interested in agricultural and veterinary work. This aspect of pharmaceutical practice is perhaps one of the least known and appreciated, although it can be both stimulating and rewarding. There is a shortage of suitably motivated pharmacists in all aspects of the manufacture and distribution of agricultural and veterinary products; consequently, the opportunities for advancement are excellent.

Before the introduction of the National Health Service (NHS) in 1948, the pharmacist was very much involved in the compounding and distribution of animal medicines, but this involvement subsequently declined. The pharmacist is the most qualified person to deal competently with drugs used for human disease and there is no obvious reason why this role should not be extended to cover the corresponding drugs used for animal diseases. In many instances, the pharmacology is the same and the properties of the products often overlap even if the brand names vary. The provisions of the Veterinary Surgeons Act 1966 prohibit the pharmacist from making any form of diagnosis of animal ailments, but there is no reason why professional judgement cannot be used to respond to symptoms described by the customer and select the appropriate medicinal product.

An additional legal category of medicine, the Pharmacy and Merchants List medicine (PML) was introduced in the early 1980s to complement those already in existence (GSL, P, and POM) under the provisions of the Medicines Act 1968. PML medicines are veterinary medicines which may be sold from pharmacies and also by agricultural merchants and saddlers registered with the Royal Pharmaceutical Society of Great Britain (RPSGB). The pharmacist is allowed to break bulk with these medicines but the saddlers and merchants are restricted to selling them in unopened containers.

The pharmacist has an important role to play in the distribution of animal medicines, but there is a need for specialist training; the NHS has developed the Diploma in Agricultural and Veterinary Pharmacy (DAgVetPharm). This course may be taken during the preregistration year. However, if the student is successful, the diploma can only be awarded after registration. Preregistration experience may be undertaken at a pharmacy that is concerned solely with the supply of agricultural and veterinary products, providing six months of the year is spent in an approved community pharmacy or hospital establishment.

A number of career prospects exist for the agricultural and veterinary pharmacist. There are specialist pharmacies that dispense veterinary prescriptions and supply items such as crop protection products, animal medicines, remedial chemicals for agricultural purposes and pest control, and animal health products.

Agricultural organisations and farmers co-operatives offer careers in general management or as advisers on animal health products. In the veterinary products industry, opportunities for the pharmacist include participation in research, development, manufacturing, and marketing activities. There are also a limited number of positions within the Ministry of Agriculture, Fisheries and Food (MAFF).

For pharmacists with appropriate specialised qualifications, it should be possible to obtain teaching appointments within veterinary schools, the Open University, and other educational establishments.

THE CIVIL SERVICE

Within the Civil Service in England, Scotland, and Wales there are currently about 100 posts held by pharmacists, although only a small number are restricted to registered pharmacists. Posts available include those relating to pharmaceutical work, for which the normal recruitment requirement is a minimum of five years' suitable experience. There are also pharmacists in scientific and administrative posts where their qualifications and experience are ideal for the particular job specification.

Department of Health, England

Pharmacists within the Pharmaceutical Division of the Department of Health in England, provide professional advice on all aspects of pharmacy practice, medicine usage, and pricing (both nationally and internationally). They also contribute to relevant aspects of NHS policy, such as pharmaceutical service provision, prescribing, the Drug Tariff, the

Selected List, the pharmaceutical industry, manpower, education, audit, and practice research.

The greatest proportion of pharmacists in the Department of Health work in the Medicines Control Agency (MCA). Pharmacists are most commonly employed as assessors to evaluate the quality aspects of data accompanying applications for licences for medicinal products. Pharmacists may also become medicines inspectors, who inspect industrial and hospital manufacturing facilities in order to ensure conformity to 'good manufacturing practice' and deal with problems involving defective medicinal products. Further opportunities exist including servicing the British Pharmacopoeia Commission (either in the secretariat or in the laboratory), working in the technical information department, or involvement with processes relating to the reclassification of medicines.

The majority of Department of Health posts require a degree of recent experience in a specialised field, although in-house training is available for some posts. A number of posts, mainly in the Medicines Control Agency, are available for people who wish to work part-time, with a degree of flexibility concerning the actual hours worked.

Scottish Office, Home and Health Department

The NHS in Scotland operates separately from the NHS in England and Wales, although there is close liaison at all levels. The Secretary of State for Scotland is responsible to Parliament for the operation of the NHS in Scotland.

The NHS in Scotland is administered by the Scottish Office Home and Health Department, which operates under the provisions of the National Health Service (Scotland) Act

1978, and the National Health Service and Community Care Act 1990. The policy divisions of the Scottish Office Home and Health Department determines NHS and Public Health Policy and the Chief Executive for the NHS in Scotland is responsible for the efficient implementation of the policy.

The Scottish Office Home and Health Department Pharmaceutical Division has as its head the Chief Pharmacist who is assisted by a deputy in providing pharmaceutical advice to the Secretary of State and to the Management Executive.

The Pharmaceutical Division undertakes a wide range of tasks. These include responsibility for the Scottish Drug Tariff, terms of service for community pharmacists, aspects of prescribing policy, and liaison with the Pharmacy Practice Division of the Common Services Agency. The Pharmacy Practice Division has responsibility for the pricing of NHS prescriptions dispensed by community pharmacists, the provision of information on the usage and costs of medicines, Scottish Prescribing Analysis for general practitioners, the Viewdata Drug Information Service (VADIS), and the Scottish Medicines Resource Centre.

There are 15 health boards in Scotland, each having responsibility for the primary care services in their area.

Welsh Office, Home and Health Department

Although the legislation referring to the NHS in Wales is the same as that for England, the operation of the service is quite separate. The Secretary of State for Wales is responsible to Parliament for its operation and the Director of the Welsh Office Health Department has responsibility for the determination of health policy and management of the service.

The Health Professionals Group, under the management of the Chief Medical Officer, provides professional advice on health matters to ministers, the Health Department, and other departments within the Welsh Office. The Health Professionals Group comprises medical, dental, scientific, environmental health and pharmaceutical divisions. It gives professional support to the health services on such issues as research, service planning, staffing, education and training, and terms and conditions of employment. The Health Professionals Group also contributes to policy on all aspects of the healthcare services.

The Pharmaceutical Division's main functions are similar to those of colleagues at the Department of Health (*see* above).

JOURNALISM AND EDITORIAL WORK

A career in journalism, medical writing, or editing can be a rewarding and exciting way of using pharmaceutical experience.

A journalist may be required to attend scientific meetings or product launches and produce a report, often to a tight deadline. The report must be interesting as well as accurate and unbiased. An 'ear' for pharmaceutical news and the ability to communicate it in a way that grabs the attention of readers are crucial. In addition, anything that is published is open to challenge; therefore evidence must be provided to support what is written.

Medical writing may involve working at a slower pace than journalism, but deadlines must still be met. For those writing for a pharmaceutical company, there may be occasions when events occur that require rapid responses, involving the production of short, sharp, press releases as well as more lengthy reports.

Technical editing does not involve working at the 'front line' all the time but can be very satisfying. Experience of drug information or clinical pharmacy can be useful but the skills acquired while training as a pharmacist provide a good background for editorial work.

Editorial work generally involves identifying, collecting, collating, evaluating, and presenting suitable material for publication; it may not involve much writing at all. When editing an article, you must have the ability to recognise the good and bad points about it. Ambiguities must be clarified, a passive verb may need to be changed to an active one, or a long sentence split into two for better comprehension. Facts must be checked, and spelling (especially of drug names and medical terms) always needs attention. Every journal has its own 'house style' and sub-editing (for example, attention to the style of headings or the presentation of tables and diagrams) is essential to ensure that the journal's distinctive style and continuity is achieved.

Writing or editorial work requires word processing abilities. These skills are usually self-taught or can sometimes be acquired on the job. Some training may be available, especially if desktop publishing is involved.

Posts for pharmaceutical editors and journalists appear in *The Pharmaceutical Journal* and in the *Chemist and Druggist*. It is also worth checking the *New Scientist* and the employment supplements in the broadsheet newspapers, especially if you are interested in the wider field of medical writing and editing.

Many of the posts advertised are office-based, full-time positions, which is not always convenient for those with family responsibilities. In addition, most editorial offices are based in London or south-east England. However, the availability of part-time editorial work is increasing, as are the opportunities to work from home.

THE PRISON PHARMACEUTICAL SERVICE

There has been a large increase in the number of prison pharmacies in recent years, creating more opportunities for pharmacists and technicians within this sector. A prison pharmacist has to possess a range of abilities; responsibilities include stock ordering, formulary work, budget management, ward rounds, clinical work, and drug identification. The pharmacy technicians employed must also adapt to the varying workload. They are sometimes left alone while the pharmacist is out on ward rounds and so have to be familiar with all operative procedures.

There are over 30 full and part-time pharmacists working in the Prison Service, based all around the country. Every pharmacist is responsible for managing the pharmaceutical service in his or her area. This can involve supplying pharmaceuticals and dressings to satellite establishments, or supervising the supply from other pharmaceutical sources.

In addition, the pharmacist is often responsible for managing the requirements of the x-ray, dental, physiotherapy, ophthalmology, and chiropody departments, including the organisation of the servicing of the equipment in these departments. Medical gases are also supplied and refilled as necessary. All first-aid cases, emergency bags, and 'riot bags' are also maintained by the pharmacy department.

There is a close working relationship between the pharmacy staff within the Prison Service and other members of the healthcare team, including medical officers, healthcare officers, physiotherapists, radiologists, dentists, and psychiatrists.

There are a number of different grades of pharmacist employed by the Prison Service. Employment is under Whitley Council terms and conditions including holiday entitlement. Before a person can take up a permanent post, checks are made on age, health, and nationality. Security checks are also carried out.

The Prison Service offers a challenging job in a somewhat unusual environment and one which allows the pharmacist to use his or her professional, organisational, and managerial skills to the full.

FURTHER INFORMATION

Bishop Y. *The Veterinary Formulary, 4th edition*. London: Pharmaceutical Press, 1998.

USEFUL ADDRESSES

**Agricultural and
Veterinary Pharmacists
Group**
Royal Pharmaceutical
Society of Great Britain
1 Lambeth High Street
London SE1 7JN
Telephone: 0171 735 9141

Department of Health
Richmond House
79 Whitehall
London
SW1A 2NS
Telephone: 0171 210 3000

**HM Prison Services
(Healthcare)**
Telephone: 0171 217 6648

Medicines Control Agency
Market Towers
1 Nine Elms Lane
London SW8 5NQ
Telephone: 0171 273 3000

NHS Confederation
Birmingham Research Park
Vincent Drive
Birmingham
West Midlands
B15 2SQ
Telephone: 0121 471 4444

10

The career break

The term 'career break' is used to describe any break from employment and applies equally to men and women. At present, most career breaks are taken by women for domestic reasons, when they need to care either for children or a dependent relative. It has been estimated that as many as 90% of these women return to work. The average time away from work for domestic reasons is now less than four years for a first child, and seven years in all to set up a family.

Generally, when a woman takes a career break, after statutory maternity leave (if applicable), she loses not only her salary but may also lose her chances of promotion. When planning a career, it is essential to consider the effects on career progression that taking a break will involve, as well as the loss of earnings.

The options for pharmacists with domestic commitments include part-time or locum work. However, such work is often professionally and financially unrewarding especially for the ambitious. There is often no career progression and it will be left to individuals to continue some form of professional updating in their own time.

Many employers may consider a pharmacist with family commitments as merely a short-term option when they need professional cover for a limited time period. The pharmacist may do locum or part-time work for many employers and not return to their previous place of employment. There is often no opportunity for continuity.

A 'career break scheme' (*see* below) offers a structured break where the employee returns to the same employer, after unpaid leave, with no loss of seniority or benefits. There is no legislation that obliges an employer to operate such a scheme but some employers now offer such a career break scheme. The increased coverage of career breaks in newspapers and in magazine articles, as well as on television and radio is heightening awareness. There is pressure for change in employment patterns and the provision of good childcare facilities.

Under the Sex Discrimination Act, industrial tribunals have ruled in individual cases that a person with domestic responsibilities who has previously worked full-time for an employer, and who has complied with the statutory declaration of intent to return to work, should be allowed to return to more flexible working arrangements (for example, to job-share or to work part-time). The European Directive on Equal Treatment complements the Sex Discrimination Act and European and United Kingdom laws apply equally to both men and women.

PREPARING FOR A CAREER BREAK

In circumstances that permit an element of choice in taking a career break, it is worthwhile spending some time on preparation and planning to ensure that you are as fully informed as possible about your choices and their implications.

Questions you should ask yourself include:

○ when is the best time in terms of my career – immediately after promotion or when I am established after promotion?

○ what duration of career break am I planning – the minimum break before returning to my current employment, a longer break but still intending to return to my current employment, or a very long break with a career change in mind?

○ how does my age affect my plans?

○ what kind of work do I want to do when I return to employment?

○ am I planning to change my employer and how will this affect my rights?

○ do I wish to work full-time upon returning to work or to work part-time?

○ are there financial considerations?

○ are there pension implications?

If planning a career break specifically for maternity leave, then some additional points will need to be considered:

○ is my career to be of equal, of more or less importance than that of my partner's and of my family responsibilities?

○ how many children, and at what intervals, am I planning to have? Will this involve taking more than one career break?

○ what sort of childcare arrangements would I prefer and who is to have responsibility for childcare? How available are childcare facilities?

When you prepare for a career break, you should consider what will happen when you return to work. If you are taking a career break for reasons other than maternity leave, you have no statutory right to return to your former employer unless you are invited to join a formal career break scheme operated by your employer.

If you are taking maternity leave, unless you are certain you want to change the direction of your career after you leave, you should arrange with your employer for your return to your original job. If, at a later date, perhaps while still on your career break, you decide against a return to your original job, you should advise your employer and you will not have lost your rights. If you have not made provision before taking a break, your employer is entitled to refuse to take you back.

In short, you are in control of your future if you say you will return before you take the break and you comply with the statutory regulations (for maternity leave) or company regulations (for maternity leave or a career break scheme) regarding periods of notification. Good communication is essential to preserve good relations with your employer.

It is imperative that you are fully aware of your rights, not only with regard to the relevant legislation but also with regard to any scheme operated by your own employer. If your employer has a career break scheme you must find out whether, on your return to work after a break, you would lose any entitlements. For instance, would it be necessary for you to work for 26 weeks after your return to work before you are once again legally protected against unfair dismissal? Would you be allowed to take another career break, and if so, how long would you have to be back at work before its commencement? Would your occupational pension rights be preserved?

CAREER BREAK SCHEMES

The objective of a career break scheme is to allow men and women to take a break from their career for an agreed length of time with the opportunity to return to the same or a similar job. The leave is unpaid and contact between the employer and employee is usually maintained, with a minimum compulsory attendance requirement to update essential skills.

The basic requirements of a career break scheme are as follows:

○ the scheme should be flexible enough to meet the needs of the organisation and its staff;

○ it must be open to both men and women;

○ it should provide opportunities for contact between employer and employee during the career break (for example, paid work sessions, 'keeping in touch' schemes, newsletters, and management bulletins). Some companies might pay the Royal Pharmaceutical Society of Great Britain (RPSGB) membership fee;

○ the scheme should provide opportunities to refresh and update skills (for example, evening meetings of social and educational value run by local branches of the RPSGB or the Guild of Hospital Pharmacists, Centre for Pharmacy Postgraduate Education distance learning courses and workshops, or educational events run by the National Association of Women Pharmacists);

○ the scheme should allow for a period of retraining/confidence building, if required;

○ flexible working arrangements to ease return to work. Usually this is to combine career and family responsibilities;

○ recognition of employee status and therefore treatment as an internal candidate for promotion, transfer, or training;

○ the employee should be re-employed on terms and conditions no less favourable than at the commencement of the career break;

○ the employee should be reinstated with the length of service previously accrued, to count towards service related terms of employment (for example, holiday entitlement or payment during illness);

○ the employee remains a member of the pension scheme (if there is one) even though no contributions are made during the career break.

Listed below are some further points to consider:

○ is the scheme applicable to full-time and part-time staff and at all grades?

○ is there a minimum length of service requirement?

○ is there a restriction on, or qualifying reason for, eligibility (for example, childcare, care of the elderly, adoption, further education, community service)? In June 1990, the Health Minister announced career breaks of up to five years for National Health Service staff in the hospital service, eligibility being restricted to those starting a family or caring for relatives. Exact details of the scheme and its implementation is decided by each individual health authority or trust;

○ is there a minimum or maximum length of time for the career break?

○ can more than one break be taken?

○ is it possible to take a part-time career break?

○ how much notice must be given of an intention to return from a career break?

○ can staff return at any time during the agreed break, if financial circumstances necessitate this?

○ must re-employment commence within a specified number of years before retirement?

○ can the employee make up pension contributions if in a company scheme?

○ is there a minimum/maximum compulsory attendance requirement? There might also be opportunities for an employee to provide temporary cover as a locum to the mutual benefit of the employer and the employee (especially if there is an agreement that during the break the employee cannot work for anyone else);

○ who will be responsible for 'keeping in touch' arrangements?

○ can benefits such as company cars, loans, and accommodation be retained whilst on a career break?

○ a career break is only one element of a work and family package. Does the employer have other family support policies (for example, family leave when children are unwell, job-share, childcare vouchers)?

MAINTAINING AWARENESS

In order to keep up-to-date with changes in the profession, arrange for professional journals to be forwarded to your home. If possible, remain a member of the RPSGB; there is a reduced membership fee for members who work less than the equivalent of 13 weeks of the year. This will enable you to receive *The Pharmaceutical Journal* and information about courses in your area run by the Centres for Pharmacy Postgraduate Education. In addition, you will have access to Society information and contact with other members of your profession through your local branch of the RPSGB.

11

Returning to work

Before returning to employment, consideration must be given to the need for re-training, the amount of flexibility required with regard to working arrangements, and the care of children during working hours.

TRAINING

Continuing education

Workshops and courses sponsored by the health departments of England, Scotland, Wales, and Northern Ireland are available. No fees are payable and community pharmacists are eligible to claim travel expenses and, where appropriate, subsistence allowances. Pharmacists who are not currently practising but are intending to return to community practice are also eligible for these courses. Information is mailed directly to pharmacists from the continuing education centres.

Study days are organised by many groups including the College of Pharmacy Practice (CPP), the Hospital Pharmacists Group, the National Association of Women Pharmacists (NAWP), the United Kingdom Clinical Pharmacy Association (UKCPA), and the National Pharmaceutical Association (NPA); details are printed in *The Pharmaceutical Journal*.

The NAWP annual weekend school provides information on a particular theme. It also represents an excellent opportunity for women returners to meet and learn from women with experience of returning to work following a lengthy absence.

Return to practice courses

In England, the Centre for Pharmacy Postgraduate Education (CPPE) has a national programme of return to practice workshops. Locations vary each year and are rotated around the country to offer maximum opportunity. The format is either residential or involves attendance one day a week for several weeks. The CPPE scheme also includes a practice attachment and applicants for the workshops are supplied with a directory of placements. The appropriate centre should be contacted for details of arrangements in Scotland, Wales, and Northern Ireland. An interactive video package has been developed by the CPPE in England and it is offered on a loan basis.

Distance learning

An extensive programme of government sponsored distance learning materials is available in England, Scotland, Wales, and Northern Ireland and full details can be obtained by writing to the relevant centre. Printed workbooks are available on a range of topics including many clinical and disease areas. Computer-assisted learning is available in England, Wales, and Scotland. The Welsh Centre holds an extensive video library for pharmacists in Wales. Pharmacists throughout Great Britain can use the Audio Visual Loan Service based at the Royal Pharmaceutical Society of Great Britain

(RPSGB). The RPSGB library offers a postal loan service. For more details, contact the librarian directly at the RPSGB.

FLEXIBLE WORKING ARRANGEMENTS

The traditional pattern of continually working a set seven or eight hours a day for five days each week between finishing education and retirement is not possible for men or women who wish, or are forced by necessity, to take an active part in bringing up a family or caring for a dependent relative.

The choice of working pattern after a career break will not only depend on your own domestic arrangements but also on the willingness of your employer, or prospective employer, to allow flexible working arrangements.

Part-time work

The need for organisations to be more competitive and flexible has in recent years resulted in dramatic changes to traditional terms of employment with temporary working, teleworking, or part-time working becoming commonplace. Historically, part-time workers may have been disadvantaged within an organisation although this is now generally not the case and an increasing proportion of the workforce in the UK is now employed on a part-time basis.

Under the terms of the Employment Protection (Part-Time Employees) Regulations 1995, part-time employees, irrespective of the number of hours per week they work, are entitled to the same rights as full-time employees. The following rights apply to all employees after two years' continuous employment and include:

○ statutory notice period of notice after four weeks;

○ protection against unfair dismissal;

○ statutory redundancy pay;

○ itemised pay statement;

○ written terms and conditions of employment;

○ rights to extended maternity absence;

○ public duties leave;

○ written reasons for dismissal.

Job-sharing

Job-sharing may be defined as the sharing of one full-time job divided between two permanent employees with joint management responsibility for that job. The salary and benefits are divided between the sharers *pro rata*. It improves the quality and availability of part-time work for people who cannot or do not want to work full-time because of other commitments.

Job-sharing can offer the opportunity to use skills and experience in a rewarding job without full-time commitment, to balance work with other important aspects of life, and it also encourages mutual support between the job-sharing partners.

The employer also benefits as two sets of skills and experience are brought to the job, the level of enthusiasm is doubled compared to a single full-time employee, and there may be more potential for flexible cover at peak periods, holiday seasons, and when domestic emergencies occur.

When establishing a job-share position, the following points should be considered:

○ recruitment: two individuals may apply as a job-share partnership or the employer may select and match successful candidates;

○ selection: this is based on the same criteria as for any job. However, the interviewers must also assess the ability of the prospective sharers to work together successfully;

○ organisation of time: this may be dictated by the job or agreed between the sharers;

○ delegation: areas of responsibility will be dependent on the needs of the job and the skills and experience of the two individual sharers;

○ contract of employment: separate, written contracts must be prepared for each individual with a *pro rata* share of salary and benefits and job description. The contract does not have to be too rigid and can usually be adjusted to meet the occasional emergency. Non-statutory occupational benefits, which are given to full-time staff, should be extended to job-sharers. These could include pension schemes, company sick pay, profit sharing, and bonuses, as well as eligibility to private health schemes.

The results of a questionnaire distributed by the NAWP showed that job-sharing was one of the most popular flexible work options. However, although there are some good role models available, difficulties may be encountered in the early stages of a partnership. Pitfalls include incompatibility between the personalities of the sharers, the day-to-day practicalities of the job, and the parameters of responsibility where decision-making is involved. The other staff have to be aware of the areas of responsibility of each sharer so that they know to whom to refer and on which matters.

Good communication is vital between sharers, employer, colleagues, and the rest of the organisation. It may be appropriate to split managerial tasks, such as appraisal sessions, so that managed staff have continuity. It is essential that mutual trust and respect exist between individuals.

Job-sharing may make it easier for women to return to work after maternity leave and so increase the use of maternity leave provisions. It can reduce staff turnover, recruitment and training costs, and make it possible to employ talented people who are not available for full-time work.

In summary, the elements of a good job-share scheme are:

○ it must be open to men and women;

○ each sharer should have a written contract of employment and job description to avoid any misunderstandings;

○ *pro rata* entitlement to the same pay and conditions as full-time employees;

○ non-statutory, occupational benefits, which are given to full-time staff, should be extended (for example, pension schemes, company sick pay, profit sharing, and discounts);

○ equal access to training and promotion;

○ the right to return to full-time work after a period of job-sharing;

○ if one sharer resigns, the option of accepting the post full-time should be made available to the other sharer.

Further points to consider:

○ consideration must be given to the nature of the post, the wishes of the sharers and the protection of their employment rights;

○ some overlap in work pattern is desirable, either as a communications time, for interviewing staff, or to provide extra cover at a peak period;

○ if one sharer is absent, the other should have the option to provide cover or not;

○ there may be contractual limitations on the job-sharers taking outside paid employment (or another post within the same organisation);

○ check how overtime, performance targets, job evaluation, allowances and bonuses are applied to job-sharers;

○ job-sharing is only one element of a work and family package. There may be other family support policies available (for example, family leave or career break schemes).

CHILDCARE

Arranging childcare can be fraught with difficulty. Even when children are school age, there is the period between the end of the school day and the end of the working day to be covered, unless you or your partner work part-time.

Crèches and nurseries are not yet widely available and some local authorities limit the time that children under the age of three may spend in crèches. It is generally accepted that there is tremendous scope for improvement in childcare services for employed parents in Great Britain, particularly as more mothers are returning to the workforce. Most people use childminders, relatives, au pairs, nannies, or mother's helps, depending on how much they can afford, how big their house is, and how many children are involved.

Childminders

A childminder may be found by looking in the local paper, on the health centre or clinic notice-boards, asking around at local playgroups, and by word of mouth. The local council will also have a list of approved childminders and will supply a list of names. Some childminders are unwilling to take babies under a year old and they should not be looking after more than three children under the age of eight years old, including their own.

Childminders must be registered with the local authority if they intend caring for children under the age of five. This registration is the childminder's safeguard. It is illegal for an unregistered person to be paid to look after a child, other than a close relation, in their own house for more than two hours.

The National Childminding Association sets minimum guidelines for pay and conditions for childminders and have produced two leaflets entitled *How to Find a Childminder* and *Pay and Conditions Advisory Leaflet.*

Nannies, au pairs, and mother's helps

If you have a large enough house, a live-in nanny or au pair is a possibility. Even if not, it may be possible to find a shared or 'live-out' nanny. Au pairs are cheaper but need to live in as one of the family; in effect, you are taking on a very young adult who may have no experience with small children and who will need considerable help in finding their way around. Mother's helps are less qualified than nannies; they may be more flexible with regards to involvement with household chores.

Nannies are specifically trained to look after children and they do not help in the house with general cleaning and ironing. It is very important that nannies are treated fairly in terms of wages, holidays, and hours. A resentful nanny is not going to stay long and there is then the problem of finding a replacement, often at short notice.

A nanny's wage will depend on where you live and the nanny's experience and qualifications; current rates are obtainable from agencies. It is normal for a nanny to work approximately 40 hours per week and to have four weeks' holiday per year plus Bank Holidays. It is essential that their National Insurance and tax are paid to protect their rights to unemployment benefit and sick pay.

Parents at Work (previously the Working Mothers' Association) produces several free factsheets, including one called *Nannies and Mother's Helps*, and also has a draft contract available for purchase. To find a nanny, an agency may be used, or an advertisement may be placed in relevant publications (for example, *Nursery World*) or the local paper. Alternatively, writing directly to a college that offers a National Nursery Examination Board (NNEB) course can be fruitful.

Day nurseries

These can be found by contacting your council social services department with whom the nursery should be registered. Day nurseries include community nurseries (open to the public but in high demand), nurseries run by the social services (intended only to serve families in dire need), and private nurseries. In all, demand exceeds the number of available places and you must get the child's name on their lists as soon as possible.

'Kids Clubs'

This is the name of a national organisation which has been founded to co-ordinate and campaign for after-school and holiday play schemes. Although some voluntary schemes operate in community centres and youth clubs, they are very few in number. Advice on starting a scheme may be obtained from 'Kids Clubs'.

Emergency planning

Unfortunately, even the happiest childcare arrangements may break down occasionally. In extreme circumstances, either you or your partner will have to take a day off work unless there is a close friend who is willing to help out in an emergency. It is worth cultivating friendships at ante-natal classes as this also provides your children with a pool of friends of the same age nearby to play with and start school together. You may consider joining the Working Mothers' Association which, in addition to being a national lobby, has local support groups and networks.

'CHILDCARE VOUCHERS'

'Childcare Vouchers' is a personalised voucher system that enables companies to contribute financially to the cost of their employee's childcare. The employer gives these vouchers to the employee, who uses them to pay only towards the cost of childcare. 'Childcare Vouchers' will draw up a contract with the childcare provider and arrange for them to be paid following receipt of the vouchers. The vouchers can be used for children from birth to 14 years of age and the employee can choose the provider, who may be a relative. 'Childcare Vouchers' offers a childcare facilities advice line and also provides an information pack. The vouchers are exempt from National Insurance and pension contributions but are currently a taxable benefit.

FURTHER INFORMATION

Pilia I. *Working Parents Survival Guide*. London: Ward Lock, 1997.

USEFUL ADDRESSES

Central Bureau
for Educational
Visits and
Exchanges
Seymour Mews
London
W1H 9PE
Telephone: 0171 486 5101

Centre for Pharmacy
Postgraduate Education
(CPPE)
School of Pharmacy and
Pharmaceutical Sciences
University of Manchester
Oxford Road
Manchester M13 9PL
Telephone: 0161 275 2324

Childcare Vouchers Ltd
(A Subsidiary of Luncheon
Vouchers Ltd)
50 Vauxhall Bridge Road
London SW1V 2RS
Telephone: 0171 834 6666

**College of Pharmacy
Practice**
University of Warwick
Science Park
Barclays Venture Centre
Coventry
West Midlands CV4 7EZ
Telephone 01203 692400

**Continuing
Pharmaceutical Education
(Northern Ireland)**
Castle Buildings
Stormont
Belfast BT4 3RA
Telephone: 01232 523 279
(Contact: Dr N Morrow)

Kids Clubs
279–281 Whitechapel
Road
London E1 1BY
Telephone: 0171 247 3009

Nannies Incorporated
63–64 Margaret Street
London W1N 7FJ
Telephone: 0171 323 3338

**National Association of
Women Pharmacists
(NAWP)**
c/o The Office Manager
Royal Pharmaceutical
Society of Great Britain
1 Lambeth High Street
London SE1 7JN
Telephone: 0171 735 9141

**National Childcare
Campaign**
Wesley House
Wild Court
London
WC2B 5AU
Telephone: 0171 405 5617

**National Childminding
Association**
8 Mason's Hill
Bromley
Kent BR2 9EY
Telephone: 0181 464 6164

New Ways to Work
309 Upper Street
London
N1 2TY
Telephone: 0171 226 4026

Nursery World
The School House
Workshop
51 Calthorpe Street
London
WC1X 0HH

Parents at Work
Murray House
Beech Street
London EC2Y 8AD
Telephone: 0171 628 3578

Royal Pharmaceutical
Society of Great Britain
Library
1 Lambeth High Street
London SE1 7JN
Telephone: 0171 735 9141

Royal Pharmaceutical
Society of Great Britain
Audio Visual Service
(Room 403)
1 Lambeth High Street
London SE1 7JN
Telephone: 0171 735 9141
Ext 288

Scottish Centre for
Postgraduate Pharmacy
Education (SCPPE)
Department of Pharmacy
University of Strathclyde
Royal College
204 George Street
Glasgow G1 1XW
Telephone: 0141 552 4400
Ext 4273/4

Welsh Centre for
Pharmacy Postgraduate
Education (WCPPE)
8 North Road
Cardiff CF1 3DY
Telephone: 01222 874784

12

Maternity leave

There is no requirement in law for women to return to work after their maternity leave period has expired. However, if employers offer more than the legal minimum, in order to retain staff, then a return to work may be a condition for eligibility for some, or all, of the enhanced benefits. The Industrial Relations Review and Report Survey has shown that women who work for organisations that offer better maternity provision are twice as likely to return to work after their maternity leave as those where only statutory leave and pay are provided.

MATERNITY BENEFITS

The Maternity Alliance issues a leaflet entitled *Pregnant at Work*, which explains fully your legal pay (Statutory Maternity Pay, SMP), maternity allowance, and other benefits. Your employer or personnel department will be able to tell you if the maternity rights where you work are better than the legal minimum requirements.

Rules and scales of payment are liable to change and it is advisable to check with your local Department of Social Security (DSS) office for the current amounts and information.

Statutory Maternity Pay

If you have worked for the same employer for at least 26 weeks and pay National Insurance contributions, you will qualify for SMP from your employer. You can claim SMP for up to a maximum of 18 weeks, starting at any time from the eleventh week before the baby is due. Some employers, for example, the National Health Service and some universities will not allow you to work beyond eleven weeks before the baby is due.

In order to qualify for SMP, the following conditions apply:

○ you must have worked for your employer for at least 26 weeks by the end of the fifteenth week before the baby is due (this week is called the qualifying week);

○ your average weekly earnings in the last eight weeks must have been at or above the amount where you start paying National Insurance contributions;

○ you must work during the qualifying week;

○ your pregnancy must last until the eleventh week before the baby is due or your baby must be born live before then;

○ you must give your employers 21 days' notice in writing and provide a Mat B1 certificate which is available from your doctor or midwife.

There are two rates of SMP, which are now payable to all women who have worked for at least 26 weeks for the same employer and who pay National Insurance contributions. The higher rate of 90% of normal earnings is paid for the first six weeks of maternity leave. The lower rate is paid for up to 12 further weeks and is paid at a rate equivalent to the higher rate of Statutory Sick Pay.

These payments are the minimum required by law for an employer to pay but some employers may be more generous.

There is no requirement to return to work after receiving SMP and there is also no requirement to repay any SMP if you do not return to work.

If any employer pays more than the minimum there may be a stipulation that some of the additional maternity pay be repaid if you choose not to return to work.

Maternity Allowance

If you do not qualify for SMP because you are self-employed, because you stop work or change jobs early in pregnancy, or because you gave notice to claim SMP too late, you may be able to claim Maternity Allowance instead. Check with your local Benefits Agency.

To qualify for Maternity Allowance, the following conditions apply:

○ you must have worked and paid standard National Insurance contributions as an employee or self-employed person for at least 26 of the 52 weeks ending with the qualifying week;

○ your pregnancy must last until the eleventh week before the baby is due.

If you have worked as a locum for an agency for some time, but not necessarily continuously, for the last 26 weeks, you may still be entitled to claim SMP. Anyone working for a hospital that has recently become a trust hospital may also be eligible for SMP. In these cases, check with your local Benefits Agency.

Maternity Allowance can be paid over the same period as SMP by the Benefits Agency; you can get the relevant forms from either your doctor or midwife. If you do not qualify for

either SMP or Maternity Allowance you may be able to claim
Statutory Sick Pay or Sickness Benefit.

Employment rights

In addition to the SMP, expectant mothers in employment are
entitled to:

○ attend ante-natal appointments without loss of pay;

○ complain of unfair dismissal because of pregnancy;

○ return to work with her employer after a period of absence on
account of pregnancy or confinement;

○ retain all contractual rights, excluding pay, for the first 14
weeks of maternity leave;

○ continue to receive normal holiday entitlement for the first 14
weeks of maternity leave.

These rights are not available to the self-employed, members
of the armed services, and other categories. The statutory
rights are minimum and do not affect the position where there
are better provisions in an employee's contract.

Ante-natal care

An expectant mother has the right to be given paid time off
for ante-natal care. You may have to produce evidence of
pregnancy and the ante-natal appointment card. All women
are entitled to free dental care and free prescriptions during
pregnancy and for one year after the baby's birth. Additional
benefits are available to women on Income Support or Family
Credit.

UNFAIR DISMISSAL

All women may now claim unfair dismissal irrespective of length of service if the dismissal is in any way connected with the pregnancy or they have recently given birth.

RETURN TO WORK

All women have the right to maternity leave for 14 weeks irrespective of length of service. Those who have two years' service 11 weeks before the expected week of confinement have the right to take maternity leave from up to 11 weeks before the expected week of confinement and up to 29 weeks after the birth.

To claim this right, you must inform your employer of the following, in writing, at least 21 days before you start maternity leave:

○ that you will be absent from work to have a baby;

○ that you intend to return to work after your absence;

○ the expected week of your confinement (a Mat B1 certificate may be requested by your employer);

○ the proposed date of return to work.

ADOPTIVE PARENTS' LEAVE

The Industrial Relations Review Report Survey in 1987 indicated that a lack of provision for leave for an adoptive parent may be discriminatory against women who are unable to conceive, but who are given the chance to adopt. There certainly seems to be no harm in asking for such leave as many employers in the smaller companies, who do not offer formal schemes, would be sympathetic to such a request. Whether the leave would be paid or unpaid would have to be negotiated on an individual basis. UK legislation on adoptive parental leave is likely to be implemented in the future.

SUMMARY

In summary, the following points should be considered by women qualifying for maternity leave:

○ it is essential to comply with the time limits and procedures to obtain SMP or Maternity Allowance;

○ does the employer provide more than the statutory maternity provisions as outlined above?

○ if more than the legal minimum is provided, is eligibility for the various beneficial elements conditional on a return to work?

○ if the employer provides a pension scheme, does unpaid maternity leave count for pension purposes? The Social Security laws provide that only paid maternity leave counts towards service for pension purposes;

○ do periods of paid and unpaid maternity leave count as service when calculating holiday entitlement?

○ can benefits such as loans, company cars, and accommodation be retained during maternity leave?

○ is there help with childcare facilities?

○ are there flexible work arrangements after maternity leave?

○   are adoptive parents entitled to any leave?

○   is there any paternity leave?

○   are there any other family support policies?

FURTHER INFORMATION

General advice on social security benefits or National Insurance may be obtained by calling *Freeline Social Security*: 0800 666555.

Local Citizens' Advice Bureaux are able to answer most queries or put you in contact with the right people.

The following booklets are available from the Benefits Agency:

FB8 *Babies and Benefits*

FB2 *Which Benefit?*

The following booklets are available from the Department of Trade and Industry:

PL710 *Employment Rights for the Expectant Mother* and *Maternity Rights: A Guide for Employers and Employees.*

USEFUL ADDRESSES

Benefits Agency
Quarry House
Quarry Hill
Leeds LS2 7UA
Telephone: 0113 232 4000

Maternity Alliance
15 Britannia Street
London WC1X 9JP

National Council for Civil Liberties (NCCL)
Women's Rights Unit
21 Tabard Street
London SE1 4LA
Telephone: 0171 403 3888

Index